My Diabetic Cookbook

50 Tasty & Delicious Recipes to Follow Your Diabetic Diet with Taste

Valerie Blanchard

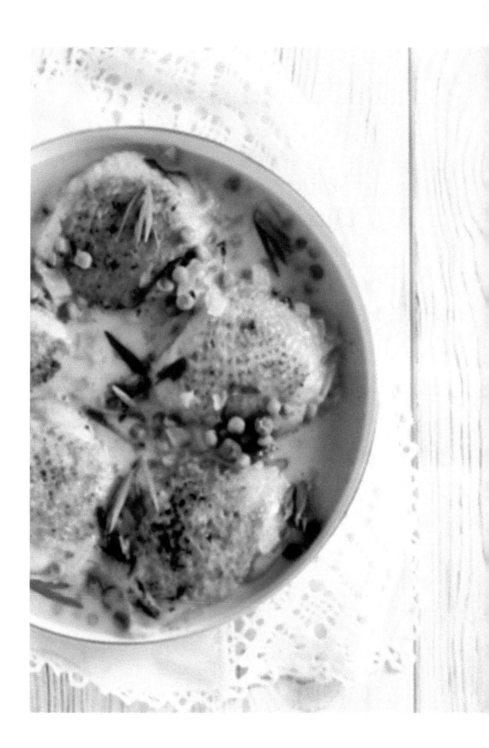

Table of Contents

6

Roasted Asparagus and Red Peppers

**Preparation Time**: 5 minutes

**Cooking Time:** 15 minutes

Serving: *4*

Ingredients:

- 1-pound (454 g) asparagus
- 2 red bell peppers, seeded
- 1 small onion
- 2 tablespoons Italian dressing

Directions:

1. Ready oven to (205ºC). Wrap baking sheet with parchment paper and set aside.
2. Combine the asparagus with the peppers, onion, dressing in a large bowl, and toss well.
3. Arrange the vegetables on the baking sheet and roast for about 15 minutes. Flip the vegetables with a spatula once during cooking.

4. Transfer to a large platter and serve.

Nutrition: 92 Calories; 10.7g Carbohydrates; 4g Fiber

Tarragon Spring Peas

Preparation Time: 10 minutes

Cooking Time: 12 minutes

Serving: 6

Ingredients:

- 1 tablespoon unsalted butter
- ½ Vidalia onion
- 1 cup low-sodium vegetable broth
- 3 cups fresh shelled peas
- 1 tablespoon minced fresh tarragon

Directions:

1. Cook butter in a pan at medium heat.
2. Sauté the onion in the melted butter for about 3 minutes, stirring occasionally.

3. Pour in the vegetable broth and whisk well. Add the peas and tarragon to the skillet and stir to combine.

4. Reduce the heat to low, cover, cook for about 8 minutes more, or until the peas are tender.

5. Let the peas cool for 5 minutes and serve warm.

Nutrition: 82 Calories; 12g Carbohydrates; 3.8g Fiber

Butter-Orange Yams

Preparation Time: 7 minutes

Cooking Time: 45 minutes

Serving: *8*

Ingredients:

- 2 medium jewel yams
- 2 tablespoons unsalted butter
- Juice of 1 large orange
- 1½ teaspoons ground cinnamon
- ¼ teaspoon ground ginger
- ¾ teaspoon ground nutmeg
- 1/8 teaspoon ground cloves

Directions:

1. Set oven at 180ºC.
2. Arrange the yam dices on a rimmed baking sheet in a single layer. Set aside.

3. Add the butter, orange juice, cinnamon, ginger, nutmeg, and garlic cloves to a medium saucepan over medium-low heat. Cook for 3 to 5 minutes, stirring continuously.

4. Spoon the sauce over the yams and toss to coat well.

5. Bake in the prepared oven for 40 minutes.

6. Let the yams cool for 8 minutes on the baking sheet before removing and serving.

Nutrition: 129 Calories; 24.7g Carbohydrates; 5g Fiber

Garlicky Mushrooms

Preparation Time: 10 minutes

Cooking Time: 12 minutes

Serving: 4

Ingredients:

- 1 tablespoon butter
- 2 teaspoons extra-virgin olive oil
- 2 pounds button mushrooms
- 2 teaspoons minced fresh garlic
- 1 teaspoon chopped fresh thyme

Directions:

1. Warm up butter and olive oil in a huge skillet over medium-high heat.

2. Add the mushrooms and sauté for 10 minutes, stirring occasionally.

3. Stir in the garlic and thyme and cook for an additional 2 minutes.

4. Season and serve on a plate.

Nutrition: 96 Calories; 8.2g Carbohydrates; 1.7g Fiber

Green Beans in Oven

__Preparation Time:__ 5 minutes

__Cooking Time:__ 17 minutes

Serving: *3*

Ingredients:

- 12 oz. green bean pods
- 1 tbsp. olive oil
- 1/2 tsp. onion powder
- 1/8 tsp. pepper
- 1/8 tsp. salt

Directions:

1. Preheat oven to 350°F. Mix green beans with onion powder, pepper, and oil.
2. Spread the seeds on the baking sheet.
3. Bake 17 minutes or until you have a delicious aroma in the kitchen.

Nutrition: 37 Calories ; 1.4g Protein; 5.5g Carbohydrates

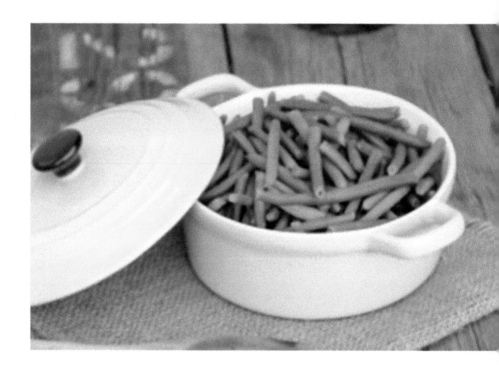

Parmesan Broiled Flounder

Preparation Time: 10 minutes

Cooking Time: 7 minutes

Serving: 2

Ingredients:

- 2 (4-oz) flounder
- 1,5 tbsp Parmesan cheese
- 1,5 tbsp mayonnaise
- 1/8 tsp soy sauce
- 1/4 tsp chili sauce
- 1/8 tsp salt-free lemon-pepper seasoning

Directions:

1. Preheat flounder.
2. Mix cheese, reduced-fat mayonnaise, soy sauce, chili sauce, seasoning.

3. Put fish on a baking sheet coated with cooking spray, sprinkle with salt and pepper.

4. Spread Parmesan mixture over flounder.

5. Broil 6 to 8 minutes or until a crust appears on the fish.

Nutrition: 200 Calories; 17g Fat; 7g Carbohydrate

Fish with Fresh Tomato - Basil Sauce

Preparation Time: 10 minutes

Cooking Time: 15 minutes

Serving*: 2*

Ingredients:

- 2 (4-oz) tilapia fillets
- 1 tbsp fresh basil, chopped
- 1/8 tsp salt
- 1 pinch of crushed red pepper
- 1 cup cherry tomatoes, chopped
- 2 tsp extra virgin olive oil

Directions:

1. Preheat oven to 400°F.
2. Arrange rinsed and patted dry fish fillets on foil (coat a foil baking sheet with cooking spray).
3. Sprinkle tilapia fillets with salt and red pepper.

4. Bake 12 - 15 minutes.

5. Meanwhile, mix leftover Ingredients in a saucepan.

6. Cook over medium-high heat until tomatoes are tender.

7. Top fish fillets properly with tomato mixture.

Nutrition: 130 Calories; 30g Protein; 1g Carbohydrates

Baked Chicken

Preparation Time: 15 minutes

Cooking Time: 25 minutes

Serving: *4*

Ingredients:

- 2 (6-oz) bone-in chicken breasts

- 1/8 tsp salt

- 1/8 tsp pepper

- 3 tsp extra virgin olive oil

- 1/2 tsp dried oregano

- 7 pitted kalamata olives

- 1 cup cherry tomatoes

- 1/2 cup onion

- 1 (9-oz) pkg frozen artichoke hearts

- 1 lemon

Directions:

1. Preheat oven to 400°F.

2. Sprinkle chicken with pepper, salt, and oregano.

3. Heat oil, add chicken and cook until it browned.

4. Place chicken in a baking dish. Arrange tomatoes, coarsely chopped olives, and onion, artichokes and lemon cut into wedges around the chicken.

5. Bake 20 minutes or until chicken is done and vegetables are tender.

Nutrition: 160 Calories; 3g Fat; 1g Carbohydrates

Seared Chicken with Roasted Vegetables

Preparation Time: 20 minutes

Cooking Time: 30 minutes

Serving: *1*

Ingredients:

- 1 (8-oz) boneless, skinless chicken breasts
- 3/4 lb. small Brussels sprouts
- 2 large carrots
- 1 large red bell pepper
- 1 small red onion
- 2 cloves garlic halved
- 2 tbsp extra virgin olive oil
- 1/2 tsp dried dill
- 1/4 tsp pepper
- 1/4 tsp salt

Directions:

1. 1.Preheat oven to 425°F.

2. Match Brussels sprouts cut in half, red onion cut into wedges, sliced carrots, bell pepper cut into pieces and halved garlic on a baking sheet.

3. Sprinkle with 1 tbsp oil and with 1/8 tsp salt and 1/8 tsp pepper. Bake until well-roasted, cool slightly.

4. In the Meantime, sprinkle chicken with dill, remaining 1/8 tsp salt and 1/8 tsp pepper. Cook until chicken is done. Put roasted vegetables with drippings over chicken.

__Nutrition:__ 170 Calories; 7g Fat; 12g Protein

Fish Simmered in Tomato-Pepper Sauce

Preparation Time: 5 minutes

Cooking Time: 10 minutes

Serving: *2*

Ingredients:

- 2 (4-oz) cod fillets
- 1 big tomato
- 1/3 cup red peppers (roasted)
- 3 tbsp almonds
- 2 cloves garlic
- 2 tbsp fresh basil leaves
- 2 tbsp extra virgin olive oil
- 1/4 tsp salt
- 1/8 tsp pepper

Directions:

1. Toast sliced almonds in a pan until fragrant.

2. Grind almonds, basil, minced garlic, 1-2 tsp oil in a food processor until finely ground.

3. Add coarsely-chopped tomato and red peppers; grind until smooth.

4. Season fish with salt and pepper.

5. Cook in hot oil in a large pan over medium-high heat until fish is browned. Pour sauce around fish. Cook 6 minutes more.

Nutrition: 90 Calories; 5g Fat; 7g Carbohydrates

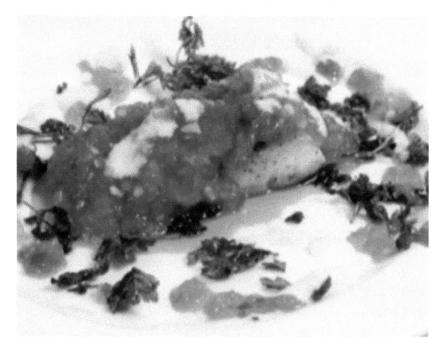

Cheese Potato and Pea Casserole

Preparation Time: 10 minutes

Cooking Time: 35 minutes

Serving: *3*

Ingredients:

- 1 tbsp olive oil
- ¾ lb. red potatoes
- ¾ cup green peas
- ½ cup red onion
- ¼ tsp dried rosemary
- ¼ tsp salt
- 1/8 tsp pepper

Directions:

1. Prepare oven to 350°F.
2. Cook 1 tsp oil in a skillet. Stir in thinly sliced onions and cook. Remove from pan.

3. Situate half of the thinly sliced potatoes and onions in bottom of skillet; top with peas, crushed dried rosemary, and 1/8 tsp each salt and pepper.

4. Place remaining potatoes and onions on top. Season with remaining 1/8 tsp salt.

5. Bake 35 minutes, pour remaining 2 tsp oil and sprinkle with cheese.

Nutrition: 80 Calories; 2g Protein; 18g Carbohydrates

Oven-Fried Tilapia

Preparation Time: 7 minutes

Cooking Time: 15 minutes

Serving: *2*

Ingredients:

- 2 (4-oz) tilapia fillets
- 1/4 cup yellow cornmeal
- 2 tbsp light ranch dressing
- 1 tbsp canola oil
- 1 tsp dill (dried)
- 1/8 tsp salt

Directions:

1. Preheat oven to 425°F. Brush both sides of rinsed and patted dry tilapia fish fillets with dressing.
2. Combine cornmeal, oil, dill, and salt.

3. Sprinkle fish fillets with cornmeal mixture.

4. Put fish on a prepared baking sheet.

5. Bake 15 minutes.

Nutrition: 96 Calories; 21g Protein; 2g Fat

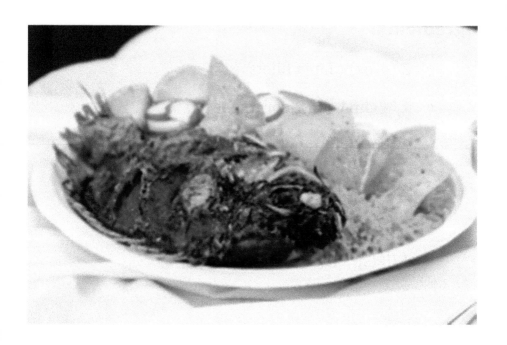

Chicken with Coconut Sauce

Preparation Time: 15 minutes

Cooking Time: 20 minutes

Serving: *2*

Ingredients:

- 1/2 lb. chicken breasts
- 1/3 cup red onion
- 1 tbsp paprika (smoked)
- 2 tsp cornstarch
- 1/2 cup light coconut milk
- 1 tsp extra virgin olive oil
- 2 tbsp fresh cilantro
- 1 (10-oz) can tomatoes and green chilis
- 1/4 cup water

Directions:

1. Cut chicken into little cubes; sprinkle with 1,5 tsp paprika.

2. Heat oil, add chicken and cook 3 to 5 minutes.

3. Remove from skillet, and fry finely-chopped onion 5 minutes.

4. Return chicken to pan. Add tomatoes,1,5 tsp paprika, and water. Bring to a boil, and then simmer 4 minutes.

5. Mix cornstarch and coconut milk; stir into chicken mixture, and cook until it has done.

6. Sprinkle with chopped cilantro.

Nutrition: 200 Calories; 13g Protein; 10g Fat

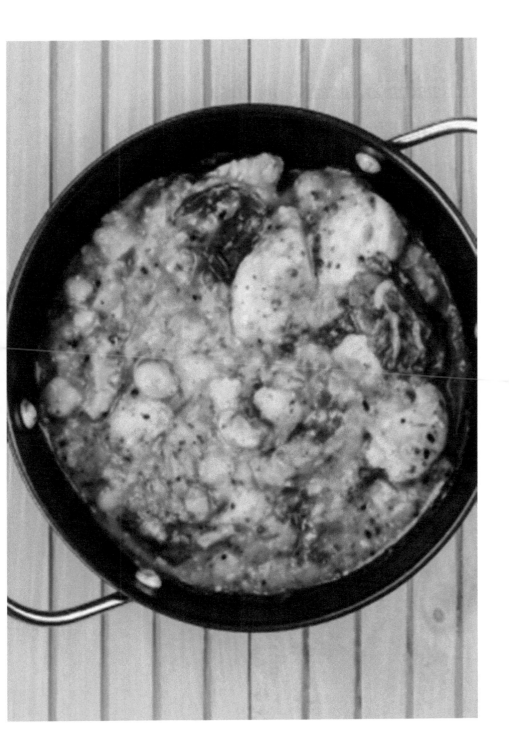

Fish with Fresh Herb Sauce

Preparation Time: 10 minutes

Cooking Time: 10 minutes

Serving: 2

Ingredients:

- 2 (4-oz) cod fillets
- 1/3 cup fresh cilantro
- 1/4 tsp cumin
- 1 tbsp red onion
- 2 tsp extra virgin olive oil
- 1 tsp red wine vinegar
- 1 small clove garlic
- 1/8 tsp salt
- 1/8 black pepper

Directions:

1. Combine chopped cilantro, finely chopped onion, oil, red wine vinegar, minced garlic, and salt.

2. Sprinkle both sides of fish fillets with cumin and pepper.

3. Cook fillets 4 minutes per side. Top each fillet with cilantro mixture.

Nutrition: 90 Calories; 4g Fat; 3g Carbohydrates

Skillet Turkey Patties

Preparation Time: 7 minutes

Cooking Time: 8 minutes

Serving*: 2*

Ingredients:

- 1/2 lb. lean ground turkey
- 1/2 cup low-sodium chicken broth
- 1/4 cup red onion
- 1/2 tsp Worcestershire sauce
- 1 tsp extra virgin olive oil
- 1/4 tsp oregano (dried)
- 1/8 tsp pepper

Directions:

1. Combine turkey, chopped onion, Worcestershire sauce, dried oregano, and pepper; make 2 patties.

2. Warm up oil and cook patties 4 minutes per side; set aside.

3. Add broth to skillet, bring to a boil. Boil 2 minutes, spoon sauce over patties.

__Nutrition:__ 180 Calories; 11g Fat; 9g Carbohydrates

Turkey Loaf

Preparation Time: 10 minutes

Cooking Time: 50 minutes

Serving: *2*

Ingredients:

- 1/2 lb. 93% lean ground turkey
- 1/3 cup panko breadcrumbs
- 1/2 cup green onion
- 1 egg
- 1/2 cup green bell pepper
- 1 tbsp ketchup
- 1/4 cup sauce (Picante)
- 1/2 tsp cumin (ground)

Directions:

1. Preheat oven to 350°F. Mix lean ground turkey, 3 tbsp Picante sauce, panko breadcrumbs, egg,

chopped green onion, chopped green bell pepper and cumin in a bowl (mix well);

2. Put the mixture into a baking sheet; shape into an oval (about 1,5 inches thick). Bake 45 minutes.

3. Mix remaining Picante sauce and the ketchup; apply over loaf. Bake 5 minutes longer. Let stand 5 minutes.

Nutrition: 161 Calories; 20g Protein; 8g Fat

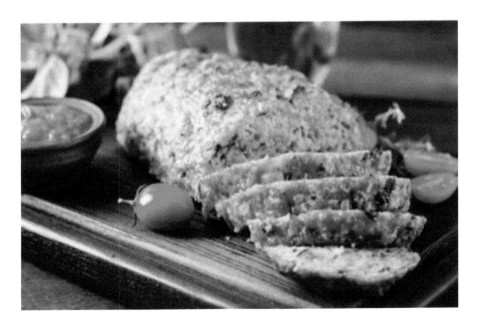

Mushroom Pasta

Preparation Time: 7 minutes

Cooking Time: 10 minutes

Serving: *4*

Ingredients:

- 4 oz whole-grain linguine
- 1 tsp extra virgin olive oil
- 1/2 cup light sauce
- 2 tbsp green onion
- 1 (8-oz) pkg mushrooms
- 1 clove garlic
- 1/8 tsp salt
- 1/8 tsp pepper

Directions:

1. Cook pasta according to package directions, drain.

2. Fry sliced mushrooms 4 minutes.

3. Stir in fettuccine minced garlic, salt and pepper. Cook 2 minutes.

4. Heat light sauce until heated; top pasta mixture properly with sauce and with finely-chopped green onion.

Nutrition: 300 Calories; 1g Fat; 15g Carbohydrates

Chicken Tikka Masala

Preparation Time: 5 minutes

Cooking Time: 15 minutes

Serving: *2*

Ingredients:

- 1/2 lb. chicken breasts
- 1/4 cup onion
- 1.5 tsp extra virgin olive oil
- 1 (14.5-oz) can tomatoes
- 1 tsp ginger
- 1 tsp fresh lemon juice
- 1/3 cup plain Greek yogurt (fat-free)
- 1 tbsp garam masala
- 1/4 tsp salt
- 1/4 tsp pepper

Directions:

1. Flavor chicken cut into 1-inch cubes with 1,5 tsp garam masala,1/8 tsp salt and pepper.

2. Cook chicken and diced onion 4 to 5 minutes.

3. Add diced tomatoes, grated ginger, 1.5 tsp garam masala, 1/8 tsp salt. Cook 8 to 10 minutes.

4. Add lemon juice and yogurt until blended.

Nutrition: 200 Calories; 26g Protein; 10g Fat

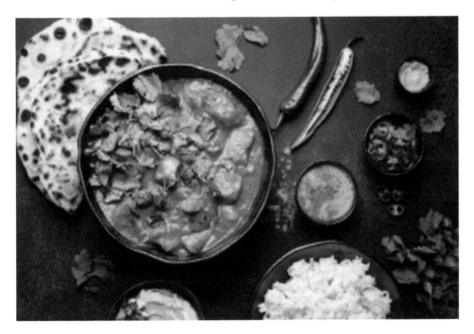

Tomato and Roasted Cod

Preparation Time: 10 minutes

Cooking Time: 35 minutes

Serving: 2

Ingredients:

- 2 (4-oz) cod fillets
- 1 cup cherry tomatoes
- 2/3 cup onion
- 2 tsp orange rind
- 1 tbsp extra virgin olive oil
- 1 tsp thyme (dried)
- 1/4 tsp salt, divided
- 1/4 tsp pepper, divided

Directions:

1. Preheat oven to 400°F. Mix in half tomatoes, sliced onion, grated orange rind, extra virgin

olive oil, dried thyme, and 1/8 salt and pepper. Fry 25 minutes. Remove from oven.

2. Arrange fish on pan, and flavor with remaining 1/8 tsp each salt and pepper. Put reserved tomato mixture over fish. Bake 10 minutes.

Nutrition: 120 Calories; 9g Protein; 2g Fat

French Broccoli Salad

Preparation Time: *10 minutes*

Cooking Time: 10 minutes

Sevings: *10*

Ingredients:

- 8 cups broccoli florets
- 3 strips of bacon, cooked and crumbled
- ¼ cup sunflower kernels
- 1 bunch of green onion, sliced

What you will need from the store cupboard:

- 3 tablespoons seasoned rice vinegar
- 3 tablespoons canola oil
- 1/2 cup dried cranberries

Directions:

1. Combine the green onion, cranberries, and broccoli in a bowl.

2. Whisk the vinegar, and oil in another bowl. Blend well.

3. Now drizzle over the broccoli mix.

4. Coat well by tossing.

5. Sprinkle bacon and sunflower kernels before serving.

Nutrition: Calories 121; Carbohydrates 14g; Cholesterol 2mg; Fiber 3g; Sugar 1g; Fat 7g; Protein 3g; Sodium 233mg

Tenderloin Grilled Salad

Preparation Time: *10 minutes*

Cooking Time: 20 minutes

Sevings: *5*

Ingredients:

- 1 lb. pork tenderloin
- 10 cups mixed salad greens
- 2 oranges, seedless, cut into bite-sized pieces
- 1 tablespoon orange zest, grated

What you will need from the store cupboard:

- 2 tablespoons of cider vinegar
- 2 tablespoons olive oil
- 2 teaspoons Dijon mustard
- 1/2 cup juice of an orange
- 2 teaspoons honey
- 1/2 teaspoon ground pepper

Directions:

1. Bring together all the dressing ingredients in a bowl.

2. Grill each side of the pork covered over medium heat for 9 minutes.

3. Slice after 5 minutes.

4. Slice the tenderloin thinly.

5. Keep the greens on your serving plate.

6. Top with the pork and oranges.

7. Sprinkle nuts (optional).

Nutrition: Calories 211; Carbohydrates 13g; Cholesterol 51mg; Fiber 3g; Sugar 0.8g; Fat 9g; Protein 20g; Sodium 113mg

Barley Veggie Salad

Preparation Time: 10 minutes

Cooking Time: 20 minutes

Sevings: 6

Ingredients:

- 1 tomato, seeded and chopped
- 2 tablespoons parsley, minced
- 1 yellow pepper, chopped
- 1 tablespoon basil, minced
- ¼ cup almonds, toasted

What you will need from the store cupboard:

- 1-1/4 cups vegetable broth
- 1 cup barley
- 1 tablespoon lemon juice
- 2 tablespoons of white wine vinegar
- 3 tablespoons olive oil
- ¼ teaspoon pepper
- 1/2 teaspoon salt

- 1 cup of water

Directions:

1. Boil the broth, barley, and water in a saucepan.
2. Reduce heat. Cover and let it simmer for 10 minutes.
3. Take out from the heat.
4. In the meantime, bring together the parsley, yellow pepper, and tomato in a bowl.
5. Stir the barley in.
6. Whisk the vinegar, oil, basil, lemon juice, water, pepper and salt in a bowl.
7. Pour this over your barley mix. Toss to coat well.
8. Stir the almonds in before serving.

Nutrition: Calories 211; Carbohydrates 27g; Cholesterol 0mg; Fiber 7g; Sugar 0g;Fat 10g; Protein 6g; Sodium 334mg

Spinach Shrimp Salad

Preparation Time: 10 minutes

Cooking Time: 10 minutes

Sevings: *4*

Ingredients:

- 1 lb. uncooked shrimp, peeled and deveined
- 2 tablespoons parsley, minced
- ¾ cup halved cherry tomatoes
- 1 medium lemon
- 4 cups baby spinach

What you will need from the store cupboard:

- 2 tablespoons butter
- 3 minced garlic cloves
- ¼ teaspoon pepper
- ¼ teaspoon salt

Directions:

1. Melt the butter over medium temperature in a nonstick skillet.
2. Add the shrimp.
3. Now cook the shrimp for 3 minutes until your shrimp becomes pink.
4. Add the parsley and garlic.
5. Cook for another minute. Take out from the heat.
6. Keep the spinach in your salad bowl.
7. Top with the shrimp mix and tomatoes.
8. Drizzle lemon juice on the salad.
9. Sprinkle pepper and salt.

__Nutrition:__ Calories 201; Carbohydrates 6g; Cholesterol 153mg; Fiber 2g; Sugar 0g; Fat 10g; Protein 21g; Sodium 350mg

Sweet Potato and Roasted Beet Salad

Preparation Time: *10 minutes*

Cooking Time: 10 minutes

Sevings: *4*

Ingredients:

- 2 beets
- 1 sweet potato, peeled and cubed
- 1 garlic clove, minced
- 2 tablespoons walnuts, chopped and toasted
- 1 cup fennel bulb, sliced

What you will need from the store cupboard:

- 3 tablespoons balsamic vinegar
- 1 teaspoon Dijon mustard
- 1 tablespoon honey
- 3 tablespoons olive oil
- ¼ teaspoon pepper
- ¼ teaspoon salt

- 3 tablespoons water

Directions:

1. Scrub the beets. Trim the tops to 1 inch.

2. Wrap in foil and keep on a baking sheet.

3. Bake until tender. Take off the foil.

4. Combine water and sweet potato in a bowl.

5. Cover. Microwave for 5 minutes. Drain off.

6. Now peel the beets. Cut into small wedges.

7. Arrange the fennel, sweet potato and beets on 4 salad plates.

8. Sprinkle nuts.

9. Whisk the honey, mustard, vinegar, water, garlic, pepper and salt.

10. Whisk in oil gradually.

11. Drizzle over the salad.

Nutrition: Calories 270; Carbohydrates 37g; Cholesterol 0mg; Fiber 6g; Sugar 0.3g; Fat 13g; Protein 5g; Sodium 309mg

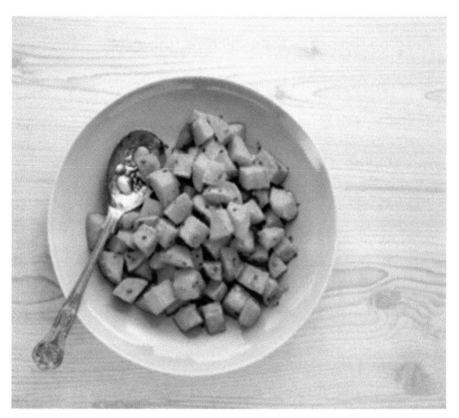

Potato Calico Salad

Preparation Time: *15 minutes*

Cooking Time: 5 minutes

Sevings: *14*

Ingredients:

- 4 red potatoes, peeled and cooked
- 1-1/2 cups kernel corn, cooked
- 1/2 cup green pepper, diced
- 1/2 cup red onion, chopped
- 1 cup carrot, shredded

What you will need from the store cupboard:

- 1/2 cup olive oil
- ¼ cup vinegar
- 1-1/2 teaspoons chili powder
- 1 teaspoon salt
- Dash of hot pepper sauce

Directions:

1. Keep all the ingredients together in a jar.

2. Close it and shake well.

3. Cube the potatoes. Combine with the carrot, onion, and corn in your salad bowl.

4. Pour the dressing over.

5. Now toss lightly.

Nutrition: Calories 146; Carbohydrates 17g; Cholesterol 0mg; Fiber 0g; Sugar 0g; Fat 9g; Protein 2g; Sodium 212mg

Mango and Jicama Salad

Preparation Time: 15 minutes

Cooking Time: 5 minutes

Sevings: *8*

Ingredients:

- 1 jicama, peeled
- 1 mango, peeled
- 1 teaspoon ginger root, minced
- 1/3 cup chives, minced
- 1/2 cup cilantro, chopped

What you will need from the store cupboard:

- ¼ cup canola oil
- 1/2 cup white wine vinegar
- 2 tablespoons of lime juice
- ¼ cup honey
- 1/8 teaspoon pepper

- ¼ teaspoon salt

Directions:

1. Whisk together the vinegar, honey, canola oil, gingerroot, paper, and salt.
2. Cut the mango and jicama into matchsticks.
3. Keep in a bowl.
4. Now toss with the lime juice.
5. Add the dressing and herbs. Combine well by tossing.

Nutrition: Calories 143; Carbohydrates 20g; Cholesterol 0mg; Fiber 3g; Sugar 1.6g; Fat 7g; Protein 1g, Sodium 78mg

Asian Crispy Chicken Salad

Preparation Time: 10 minutes

Cooking Time: 10 minutes

Sevings: *2*

Ingredients:

- 2 chicken breasts halved, skinless
- 1/2 cup panko bread crumbs
- 4 cups spring mix salad greens
- 4 teaspoons of sesame seeds
- 1/2 cup mushrooms, sliced

What you will need from the store cupboard:

- 1 teaspoon sesame oil
- 2 teaspoons of canola oil
- 2 teaspoons hoisin sauce
- ¼ cup sesame ginger salad dressing

Directions:

1. Flatten the chicken breasts to half-inch thickness.
2. Mix the sesame oil and hoisin sauce. Brush over the chicken.
3. Combine the sesame seeds and panko in a bowl.
4. Now dip the chicken mix in it.
5. Cook each side of the chicken for 5 minutes.
6. In the meantime, divide the salad greens between two plates.
7. Top with mushroom.
8. Slice the chicken and keep on top. Drizzle the dressing.

Nutrition: Calories 386; Carbohydrates 29g; Cholesterol 63mg; Fiber 6g; Sugar 1g; Fat 17g;Protein 30g; Sodium 620mg

Kale, Grape and Bulgur Salad

Preparation Time: 10 minutes

Cooking Time: 15 minutes

Sevings: 6

Ingredients:

- 1 cup bulgur
- 1 cup pecan, toasted and chopped
- ¼ cup scallions, sliced
- 1/2 cup parsley, chopped
- 2 cups California grapes, seedless and halved

What you will need from the store cupboard:

- 2 tablespoons of extra virgin olive oil
- ¼ cup of juice from a lemon
- Pinch of kosher salt
- Pinch of black pepper
- 2 cups of water

Directions:

1. Boil 2 cups of water in a saucepan

2. Stir the bulgur in and 1/2 teaspoon of salt.

3. Take out from the heat.

4. Keep covered. Drain.

5. Stir in the other ingredients.

6. Season with pepper and salt.

Nutrition: Calories 289; Carbohydrates 33g; Fat 17g; Protein 6g; Sodium 181mg

Strawberry Salsa

Preparation Time: 10 minutes

Cooking Time: 5 minutes

Sevings: *4*

Ingredients:

- 4 tomatoes, seeded and chopped
- 1-pint strawberry, chopped
- 1 red onion, chopped
- 2 tablespoons of juice from a lime
- 1 jalapeno pepper, minced

What you will need from the store cupboard:

- 1 tablespoon olive oil
- 2 garlic cloves, minced

Directions:

1. Bring together the strawberries, tomatoes, jalapeno, and onion in the bowl.

2. Stir in the garlic, oil, and lime juice.

3. Refrigerate. Serve with separately cooked pork or poultry.

Nutrition: Calories 19; Carbohydrates 3g; Fiber 1g; Sugar 0.2g; Cholesterol 0mg; Total Fat 1g; Protein 0g

Garden Wraps

Preparation Time: 20 minutes

Cooking Time: 10 minutes

Sevings: *8*

Ingredients:

- 1 cucumber, chopped
- 1 sweet corn
- 1 cabbage, shredded
- 1 tablespoon lettuce, minced
- 1 tomato, chopped

What you will need from the store cupboard:

- 3 tablespoons of rice vinegar
- 2 teaspoons peanut butter
- 1/3 cup onion paste
- 1/3 cup chili sauce
- 2 teaspoons of low-sodium soy sauce

Directions:

1. Cut corn from the cob. Keep in a bowl.

2. Add the tomato, cabbage, cucumber, and onion paste.

3. Now whisk the vinegar, peanut butter, and chili sauce together.

4. Pour this over the vegetable mix. Toss for coating.

5. Let this stand for 10 minutes.

6. Take your slotted spoon and place 1/2 cup salad in every lettuce leaf.

7. Fold the lettuce over your filling.

Nutrition: Calories 64; Carbohydrates 13g; Fiber 2g; Sugar 1g; Cholesterol 0mg; Total Fat 1g; Protein 2g

Party Shrimp

__Preparation Time:__ 15 minutes

__Cooking Time__: 10 minutes

Sevings: *30*

Ingredients:

- 16 oz. uncooked shrimp, peeled and deveined
- 1-1/2 teaspoons of juice from a lemon
- 1/2 teaspoon basil, chopped
- 1 teaspoon coriander, chopped
- 1/2 cup tomato

What you will need from the store cupboard:

- 1 tablespoon of olive oil
- 1/2 teaspoon Italian seasoning
- 1/2 teaspoon paprika
- 1 sliced garlic clove
- ¼ teaspoon pepper

Directions:

1. Bring together everything except the shrimp in a dish or bowl.

2. Add the shrimp. Coat well by tossing. Set aside.

3. Drain the shrimp. Discard the marinade.

4. Keep them on a baking sheet. It should not be greased.

5. Broil each side for 4 minutes. The shrimp should become pink.

Nutrition: Calories 14; Carbohydrates 0g; Fiber 0g; Sugar 0g; Cholesterol 18mg; Total Fat 0g; Protein 2g

Zucchini Mini Pizzas

Preparation Time: 20 minutes

Cooking Time: 10 minutes

Sevings: *24*

Ingredients:

- 1 zucchini, cut into ¼ inch slices diagonally
- 1/2 cup pepperoni, small slices
- 1 teaspoon basil, minced
- 1/2 cup onion, chopped
- 1 cup tomatoes

What you will need from the store cupboard:

- 1/8 teaspoon pepper
- 1/8 teaspoon salt
- 3/4 cup mozzarella cheese, shredded
- 1/3 cup pizza sauce

Directions:

1. Preheat your broiler. Keep the zucchini in 1 layer on your greased baking sheet.
2. Add the onion and tomatoes. Broil each side for 1 to 2 minutes till they become tender and crisp.
3. Now sprinkle pepper and salt.
4. Top with cheese, pepperoni, and sauce.
5. Broil for a minute. The cheese should melt.
6. Sprinkle basil on top.

Nutrition: Calories 29; Carbohydrates 1g; Fiber 0g; Sugar 1g; Cholesterol 5mg; Total Fat 2g; Protein 2g

Garlic-Sesame Pumpkin Seeds

Preparation Time: 10 minutes

Cooking Time: 20 minutes

Sevings: *2*

Ingredients:

- 1 egg white
- 1 teaspoon onion, minced
- 1/2 teaspoon caraway seeds
- 2 cups pumpkin seeds
- 1 teaspoon sesame seeds

What you will need from the store cupboard:

- 1 garlic clove, minced
- 1 tablespoon of canola oil
- ¾ teaspoon of kosher salt

Directions:

1. Preheat your oven to 350 ºF.

2. Whisk together the oil and egg white in a bowl.

3. Include pumpkin seeds. Coat well by tossing.

4. Now stir in the onion, garlic, sesame seeds, caraway seeds, and salt.

5. Spread in 1 layer in your parchment-lined baking pan.

6. Bake for 15 minutes until it turns golden brown.

Nutrition: Calories 95; Carbohydrates 9g; Fiber 3g; Sugar 0g; Cholesterol 0mg; Total Fat 5g; Protein 4g

Thai Quinoa Salad

Preparation Time: 10 minutes

Cooking Time: 0 minutes

Sevings: 1-2

Ingredients:

Ingredients used for dressing:

- 1 tbsp. Sesame seed

- 1 tsp. Chopped garlic

- 1 tsp. Lemon, fresh juice

- 3 tsp. Apple Cider Vinegar

- 2 tsp. Tamari, gluten-free.

- 1/4 cup of tahini (sesame butter)

- 1 pitted date

- 1/2 tsp. Salt

- 1/2 tsp. toasted Sesame oil

Salad ingredients:

- 1 cup of quinoa, steamed
- 1 big handful of arugulas
- 1 tomato cut in pieces
- 1/4 of the red onion, diced

Directions:

1. Add the following to a small blender: 1/4 cup + 2 tbsp.

2. Filtered water, the rest of the **Ingredients** . Blend, man. Steam 1 cup of quinoa in a steamer or a rice pan, then set aside.

3. Combine the quinoa, the arugula, the tomatoes sliced, the red onion diced on a **Serving** plate or bowl, add the Thai dressing

4. and serve with a spoon.

Nutrition: Calories: 100; Carbohydrates: 12 g

Green Goddess Bowl and Avocado Cumin Dressing

Preparation Time: 10 minutes

Cooking Time: 0 minutes

Sevings: 1-2

Ingredients:

Ingredients for the dressing of avocado cumin:

- 1 Avocado
- 1 tbsp. Cumin Powder
- 2 limes, freshly squeezed
- 1 cup of filtered water
- 1/4 seconds. sea salt
- 1 tbsp. Olive extra virgin olive oil
- Cayenne pepper dash
- Optional: 1/4 tsp. Smoked pepper

Tahini Lemon Dressing Ingredients:

- 1/4 cup of tahini (sesame butter)
- 1/2 cup of filtered water (more if you want thinner, less thick)
- 1/2 lemon, freshly squeezed
- 1 clove of minced garlic
- 3/4 tsp. Sea salt (Celtic Gray, Himalayan, Redmond Real Salt)
- 1 tbsp. Olive extra virgin olive oil
- black pepper taste

Salad ingredients:

- 3 cups of kale, chopped
- 1/2 cup of broccoli flowers, chopped
- 1/2 zucchini (make spiral noodles)
- 1/2 cup of kelp noodles, soaked and drained
- 1/3 cup of cherry tomatoes, halved.
- 2 tsp. hemp seeds

Directions:

1. Gently steam the kale and the broccoli (flash the steam for 4 minutes), set aside.

2. Mix the zucchini noodles and kelp noodles and toss with a generous portion of the smoked avocado cumin dressing. Add the cherry tomatoes and stir again.

3. Place the steamed kale and broccoli and drizzle with the lemon tahini dressing. Top the kale and the broccoli with the noodles and tomatoes and sprinkle the whole dish with the hemp seeds.

Nutrition: Calories: 89; Carbohydrates: 11g; Fat: 1.2g; Protein: 4g

Sweet and Savory Salad

Preparation Time: 10 minutes

Cooking Time: 0 minutes

Sevings: 1-2

Ingredients:

- 1 big head of butter lettuce
- 1/2 of cucumber, sliced
- 1 pomegranate, seed or 1/3 cup of seed
- 1 avocado, 1 cubed
- 1/4 cup of shelled pistachio, chopped

Ingredients for dressing:

- 1/4 cup of apple cider vinegar
- 1/2 cup of olive oil
- 1 clove of garlic, minced

Directions:

1. Put the butter lettuce in a salad bowl.

2. Add the remaining ingredients and toss with the salad dressing.

Nutrition: Calories: 68; Carbohydrates: 8g; Fat: 1.2g; Protein: 2g

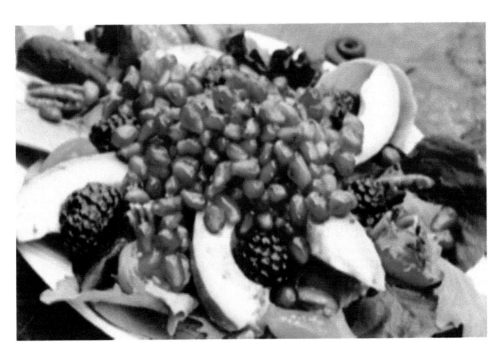

Kale Pesto's Pasta

Preparation Time: 10 minutes

Cooking Time: 0 minutes

Sevings: 1-2

Ingredients:

- 1 bunch of kale

- 2 cups of fresh basil

- 1/4 cup of extra virgin olive oil

- 1/2 cup of walnuts

- 2 limes, freshly squeezed

- Sea salt and chili pepper

- 1 zucchini, noodle (spiralizer)

- Optional: garnish with chopped asparagus, spinach leaves, and tomato.

Directions:

1. The night before, soak the walnuts in order to improve absorption.

2. Put all the recipe Ingredients in a blender and blend until the consistency of the cream is reached.

3. Add the zucchini noodles and enjoy.

Nutrition: Calories: 55; Carbohydrates: 9 g; Fat: 1.2g

Beet Salad with Basil Dressing

Preparation Time: 10 minutes

Cooking Time: 0 minutes

Sevings: *4*

Ingredients:

Ingredients for the dressing

- ¼ cup blackberries

- ¼ cup extra-virgin olive oil

- Juice of 1 lemon

- 2 tablespoons minced fresh basil

- 1 teaspoon poppy seeds

- A pinch of sea salt

- For the salad

- 2 celery stalks, chopped

- 4 cooked beets, peeled and chopped

- 1 cup blackberries

- 4 cups spring mix

Directions:

1. To make the dressing, mash the blackberries in a bowl. Whisk in the oil, lemon juice, basil, poppy seeds, and sea salt.

2. To make the salad: Add the celery, beets, blackberries, and spring mix to the bowl with the dressing.

3. Combine and serve.

Nutrition: Calories: 192; Fat: 15g; Carbohydrates: 15g; Protein: 2g

Basic Salad with Olive Oil Dressing

Preparation Time: 10 minutes

Cooking Time: *0 minute*

Sevings: *4*

Ingredients:

- 1 cup coarsely chopped iceberg lettuce
- 1 cup coarsely chopped romaine lettuce
- 1 cup fresh baby spinach
- 1 large tomato, hulled and coarsely chopped
- 1 cup diced cucumber
- 2 tablespoons extra-virgin olive oil
- ¼ teaspoon of sea salt

Directions:

1. In a bowl, combine the spinach and lettuces. Add the tomato and cucumber.

2. Drizzle with oil and sprinkle with sea salt.

3. Mix and serve.

Nutrition: Calories: 77; Fat: 4g; Carbohydrates: 3g; Protein: 1g

Spinach & Orange Salad with Oil Drizzle

Preparation Time: 10 minutes

Cooking Time: *0 minute*

Sevings: *4*

Ingredients:

- 4 cups fresh baby spinach
- 1 blood orange, coarsely chopped
- ½ red onion, thinly sliced
- ½ shallot, finely chopped
- 2 tbsp. minced fennel fronds
- Juice of 1 lemon
- 1 tbsp. extra-virgin olive oil
- Pinch sea salt

Directions:

1. In a bowl, toss together the spinach, orange, red onion, shallot, and fennel fronds.

2. Add the lemon juice, oil, and sea salt.

3. Mix and serve.

Nutrition: Calories: 79; Fat: 2g; Carbohydrates: 8g; Protein: 1g

Fruit Salad with Coconut-Lime Dressing

Preparation Time: 5 minutes

Cooking Time: 0 minutes

Sevings: *4*

Ingredients:

Ingredients for the dressing

- ¼ cup full-fat canned coconut milk

- 1 tbsp. raw honey

- Juice of ½ lime

- Pinch sea salt

- For the salad

- 2 bananas, thinly sliced

- 2 mandarin oranges, segmented

- ½ cup strawberries, thinly sliced

- ½ cup raspberries

- ½ cup blueberries

Directions :

1. To make the dressing: whisk all the dressing ingredients in a bowl.

2. To make the salad: Add the salad ingredients in a bowl and mix.

3. Drizzle with the dressing and serve.

__Nutrition__: Calories: 141; Fat: 3g; Carbohydrates: 30g; Protein: 2g

Cranberry And Brussels Sprouts With Dressing

Preparation Time: 10 minutes

Cooking Time: *0 minute*

Servings: *4*

Ingredients:

Ingredients for the dressing

- 1/3 cup extra-virgin olive oil

- 2 tbsp. apple cider vinegar

- 1 tbsp. pure maple syrup

- Juice of 1 orange

- ½ tbsp. dried rosemary

- 1 tbsp. scallion, whites only

- Pinch sea salt

For the salad

- 1 bunch scallions, greens only, finely chopped

- 1 cup Brussels sprouts, stemmed, halved, and thinly sliced
- ½ cup fresh cranberries
- 4 cups fresh baby spinach

Directions:

1. To make the dressing: In a bowl, whisk the dressing ingredients.
2. To make the salad: Add the scallions, Brussels sprouts, cranberries, and spinach to the bowl with the dressing.
3. Combine and serve.

__Nutrition:__ Calories: 267; Fat: 18g; Carbohydrates: 26g; Protein: 2g

Parsnip, Carrot, And Kale Salad with Dressing

Preparation Time: 10 minutes

Cooking Time: 0 minutes

Servings: *4*

Ingredients:

Ingredients for the dressing

- 1/3 cup extra-virgin olive oil

- Juice of 1 lime

- 2 tbsp. minced fresh mint leaves

- 1 tsp. pure maple syrup

- Pinch sea salt

For the salad

- 1 bunch kale, chopped

- ½ parsnip, grated

- ½ carrot, grated

- 2 tbsp. sesame seeds

Directions:

1. To make the dressing, mix all the dressing Ingredients in a bowl.

2. To make the salad, add the kale to the dressing and massage the dressing into the kale for 1 minute.

3. Add the parsnip, carrot, and sesame seeds.

4. Combine and serve.

Nutrition: Calories: 214; Fat: 2g; Carbohydrates: 12g; Protein: 2g

Tomato Toasts

Preparation Time: 5 minutes

Cooking Time: 5 minutes

Sevings: *4*

Ingredients:

- 4 slices of sprouted bread toasts

- 2 tomatoes, sliced

- 1 avocado, mashed

- 1 teaspoon olive oil

- 1 pinch of salt

- ¾ teaspoon ground black pepper

Directions:

1. Blend together the olive oil, mashed avocado, salt, and ground black pepper.

2. When the mixture is homogenous – spread it over the sprouted bread.

3. Then place the sliced tomatoes over the toasts.

4. Enjoy!

Nutrition: Calories: 125; Fat: 11.1g; Carbohydrates: 7.0g; Protein: 1.5g

Everyday Salad

Preparation Time : 10 minutes

Cooking Time: 40 minutes

Sevings: *6*

Ingredients:

- 5 halved mushrooms
- 6 halved Cherry (Plum) Tomatoes
- 6 rinsed Lettuce Leaves
- 10 olives
- ½ chopped cucumber
- Juice from ½ Key Lime
- 1 teaspoon olive oil
- Pure Sea Salt

Directions:

1. Tear rinsed lettuce leaves into medium pieces and put them in a medium salad bowl.

2. Add mushrooms halves, chopped cucumber, olives and cherry tomato halves into the bowl. Mix well. Pour olive and Key Lime juice over salad.

3. Add pure sea salt to taste. Mix it all till it is well combined.

Nutrition: Calories: 88; Carbohydrates: 11g; Fat: 5g; Protein: 8g

Super-Seedy Salad with Tahini Dressing

Preparation Time: 10 minutes

Cooking Time: 0 minutes

Sevings: *1-2*

Ingredients:

- 1 slice stale sourdough, torn into chunks

- 50g mixed seeds

- 1 tsp. cumin seeds

- 1 tsp. coriander seeds

- 50g baby kale

- 75g long-stemmed broccoli, blanched for a few minutes then roughly chopped

- ½ red onion, thinly sliced

- 100g cherry tomatoes, halved

- ½ a small bunch flat-leaf parsley, torn

DRESSING

- 100ml natural yogurt

- 1 tbsp. tahini

- 1 lemon, juiced

Directions:

1. Heat the oven to 200°C/fan 180°C/gas 6. Put the bread into a food processor and pulse into very rough breadcrumbs. Put into a bowl with the mixed seeds and spices, season, and spray well with oil. Tip onto a non-stick baking tray and roast for 15-20 minutes, stirring and tossing regularly, until deep golden brown.

2. Whisk together the dressing ingredients, some seasoning and a splash of water in a large bowl. Tip the baby kale, broccoli, red onion, cherry tomatoes and flat-leaf parsley into the dressing and mix well. Divide between 2 plates and top with the crispy breadcrumbs and seeds.

Nutrition: Calories: 78; Carbohydrates: 6 g; Fat: 2g; Protein: 1.5g

Vegetable Salad

Preparation Time: 10 minutes

Cooking Time: 0 minutes

Sevings: *1-2*

Ingredients:

- 4 cups each of raw spinach and romaine lettuce
- 2 cups each of cherry tomatoes, sliced cucumber, chopped baby carrots and chopped red, orange and yellow bell pepper
- 1 cup each of chopped broccoli, sliced yellow squash, zucchini and cauliflower.

Directions:

1. Wash all these vegetables.
2. Mix in a large mixing bowl and top off with a non-fat or low-fat dressing of your choice.

Nutrition: Calories: 48; Carbohydrates: 11g; Protein: 3g

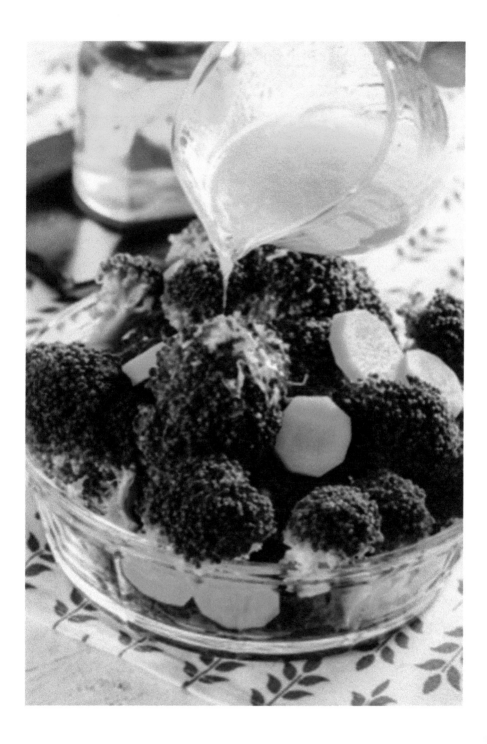

Greek Salad

Preparation Time: 10 minutes

Cooking Time: 0 minutes

Sevings: *1-2*

Ingredients:

- 1 Romaine head, torn in bits

- 1 cucumber sliced

- 1 pint cherry tomatoes, halved

- 1 green pepper, thinly sliced

- 1 onion sliced into rings

- 1 cup kalamata olives

- 1 ½ cups feta cheese, crumbled

For dressing combine:

- 1 cup olive oil

- 1/4 cup lemon juice

- 2 tsp. oregano

- Salt and pepper

Directions:

1. Lay ingredients on plate.

2. Drizzle dressing over salad

Nutrition: Calories: 107; Carbohydrates: 18g; Fat: 1.2 g;
Protein: 1g

Alkaline Spring Salad

Preparation Time: 10 minutes

Cooking Time: 0 minutes

Sevings: *1-2*

Eating seasonal fruits and vegetables is a fabulous way of taking care of yourself and the environment at the same time. This alkaline-electric salad is delicious and nutritious.

Ingredients:

- 4 cups seasonal approved greens of your choice
- 1 cup cherry tomatoes
- 1/4 cup walnuts
- 1/4 cup approved herbs of your choice

For the dressing:

- 3-4 key limes
- 1 tbsp. of homemade raw sesame

- Sea salt and cayenne pepper

Directions:

1. First, get the juice of the key limes. In a small bowl, whisk together the key lime juice with the homemade raw sesame "tahini" butter. Add sea salt and cayenne pepper, to taste.

2. Cut the cherry tomatoes in half.

3. In a large bowl, combine the greens, cherry tomatoes, and herbs. Pour the dressing on top and "massage" with your hands.

4. Let the greens soak up the dressing. Add more sea salt, cayenne pepper, and herbs on top if you wish. Enjoy!

Nutrition: Calories: 77; Carbohydrates: 11g

Lightning Source UK Ltd.
Milton Keynes UK
UKHW020643100621
385263UK00001B/216